ARE WEIGHT AND POUNDS THE SAME THING?

Cedric Milligan Sr.

Milligan Books   **California**

Published and Distributed by:
Milligan Books, Inc.
An imprint of Professional Business Consultants

Cover Design By
Clark Graphic Images

Formatting By
Alpha Desktop Publishing

First Printing, July 2002
10987654321

ISBN 0-9719749-4-2

DEDICATION

To my son, Cedric Milligan Jr.: You bring light into my life when I see darkness. Without you I don't know if I could have written this book.

To my late grandmother, Laura Milligan, for all your love.

To my late grandfather Simon Hunter, I inherited your spirit. Thank you for leading the way.

Table Of Contents

ABOUT THE AUTHOR

Cedric Milligan Sr. has had an interest in health since the age 15. He owned Herb-Life Connection 2000 Health Food store in Los Angeles.

He received an Iridologist Certificate from Dr. Paul Goss School of Iridologist. He also studied under Dr. Joyce Willoughby at The Institute of herbal Medicine.

Cedric Milligan Sr. is a personal fitness trainer and health consultant.

INTRODUCTION

ARE WEIGHT AND POUNDS THE SAME THING? What you need to know about yourself.

When it comes to wanting to know about your body, most of the time people just don't know what questions to ask or how to find out more about what's going on inside their bodies. No one is born with the skill to know everything the human body can do but GOD. He did make people that would learn about the human body so they could teach others about what the body can do, what to expect out of the body, and what makes the human body function. Well, that is where I come in.

I am one of those people here to teach you a little something about your body. What gives me the right to say what I know is the truth? As you keep reading, I will give you the facts on how some of your body organs work. You will find out how to keep your body engine going longer than the average life span in this day and time.

There are many people who can tell you something about your body but you have to ask yourself is it just their own opinion on how they think the body works, or is it the truth? There are people who know that they can make some money from telling you what is wrong with your body, and there are some who really know about the human body. If you look closely those people who always know the truth about something, the power players with the money, will try to label the herbalist as a crazy scientist or a person who doesn't know what she/he is talking about. Herbalists are natural scientists who deal with natural healing of the body. There are doctors who recommend herbs to some of their clients. The people at the top, who profit from the deaths of people, need to keep the people in the dark about what's really going on with the company or the product they have or just the information they are giving you in the first place.

When it comes to your health you have to remember that in most cases your friends do not know what they're talking about if they are not in the study of health. You always have people who want to tell you about what they took when they were sick. A cold or flu is one of your most common illnesses but you have to know what type of cold or flu you have to properly treat it. Not every one knows about the body, just like your car the average person knows nothing about what goes on under the hood of their car. That's why you go to the doctor and the auto shop, to people who have learned and studied how the car and body work. Other people can only give you their opinion, and you might end up feeling worse than before. Call the people who know best. Some people are just trying to help, but not all help is good help.

Most people need to follow their own mind and when you think someone is telling the truth, ask yourself, could this person be telling me the truth and I am just not ready for the truth?

Well, sit back and hold on because you are going down the road to the truth about your health. Believe me, I have better things to be doing with my time than writing a book about something that's not the truth. Plus I don't have a weight problem, so what good would that do for you or me?

This book will be the one book that will help change the way you think and look at your body. Well, in a few minutes you will be walking differently and talking differently, looking like, a whole new person 100% better. Get ready to come out fighting! Now you know, people are always looking for the truth. They may get tried but they keep looking until it comes their way. Now you can take better care of your body because you know how it works.

Chapter 1

What Is Weight?

Weight is something that has heaviness to it, like a box of books, bricks, etc. The main thing about weight is that you can balance out weight to an even scale. By carrying too much weight, your whole shape can just look out of place. Now it is time to do something about this new weight you are carrying around town. Your body is not looking like it used to. Clothes are not fitting the same as they used to. It is costing you more to keep up with your old style of dressing. So somewhere down the line you think you can still fit those clothes that make you feel uncomfortable. It still has not sunk deep enough in your head. Let me go ahead and shake you up a little bit. I know you're not shaking anything with those extra 55 pounds holding you down.

Now show me what you're really working with, Mr. or Ms.

"I am so cool; I am not going to let this new weight hold me from doing my thing." You can't be too cool or happy about your size if you're taking time out of your day to read this book. Something must be on your mind about the way you're really looking these days when you wake up and look at yourself in the mirror. Well, look at it this way, if you cannot keep it real with yourself, how are you going to believe I am for real? When you are not real with yourself, how can someone help you? I guess it will hit home when you come out of believing that lie that the new weight looks good on you. If the weight looks so good on you, why are you just now gaining the weight? Did it just jump out at you all at once, saying take some of this extra pound and become my new friend? I know that is not what happens, but do you know what happened?

You may be able to lie or give a silly opinion

about why you're getting bigger to fool some people but you are not fooling me because I do not even know you. So don't fool yourself, trying to impress some one. However, I know you're saying to yourself there is "nothing wrong with my weight." Well, put the book down. I don't think you can. Just because people at your job or church or even around where you live feel okay to have grown fatter and bigger by the day, that does not make it okay for you.

I have friends who are 55-100 pounds overweight; they tell me the weight doesn't bother them. As long as their mates are not complaining, it's okay. If you think that way you really need to keep on reading this book because we all know people will tell you whatever you want to hear to make you feel good. Therefore, who can you believe–yourself or other people?

Some people like large men and women just because they are big, it has nothing to do with who you are. You may think you have something going on with a person and it may be just because that person likes big women or men. Some people will leave a person if they were to try to lose some of the weight. See, that's why they wanted you in the first place. It's o.k. That is just life, so move on.

Some of the things I am talking about concerning weight may not fit every one that reads this book. Everyone's body is not the same. I say this because I know a lot of people who love to tell me that "all this fat came from when I was a baby." That's the funniest thing I have ever heard. Now I do not know what would make a person just say something like that or how they came up with that. But some people can hear something and if it sounds good to them, they believe that's the way it should be and some never think to find out if that's the truth. If you did not know already, there is no such thing as baby fat. Babies are fat when their parents feed them too much food. You are not a baby anymore.

16

What happens is that the fatty tissue in your body developed faster than your height, so the fat from the food had nowhere to go but into rolls of fat. Sometimes feeding a baby too much stops that balance of the baby's growth. Babies will grow out of body fat when you begin to feed them less food. The more food a person puts in their body, whether they're a baby or an adult, the more food, they will want, even when they're not hungry. So, keep that in mind if you plan to have kids or already have one. Let's face the fact that you're just a fat person. You need to do something about being overweight.

The fatty tissue and muscle tissue protect the bones as we grow. What happens is the extra fat you put in your body from the foods you eat has a big effect on the growth of your bones. The fatty tissue in the body helps the body grow. So does the 70% of water in the body. The foods we eat all contain some type of calories from fat as well as calories from protein, carbs, etc. If you're not having bowel

17

eliminations on a regular basis, where do you think the food is going? The fat from the food stays in the colon, making it look like you have rolls of fat. (See Fig. 1 and Fig. 2 diagram on pages 24 and 25.)

Don't just sit around wishing you could do something about your weight. Believe in yourself and stop telling yourself "I look good." You may think you look good but your body's not feeling so good with the extra pounds. The human body is only made up to take on so much extra body fat at a time before it begins to start moving some of your organs inside of the body. The only organ in your body that can hold pounds is your colon.

The colon grows 29 feet, you can put up to 300 pounds in there without it ever coming out. You still have to remember that your body is made out of fatty tissue, and muscle tissue, not pounds.

Now, I am going back just a step or two to a point I made earlier. When I said that the pounds' added pressure would begin to start moving some of your body organs, well follow me and you will understand the truth. For the people out there who have diabetes, here are some of the main reasons why. You are overweight, carrying too many extra pounds on your body that are not supposed to be there. Now you keep asking yourself "why am I having so many new problems going on inside my body?" Well, the new pounds you put on are holding you down and destroying your body organs.

The pancreas sits right behind your large colon. Once you start to put pounds in your colon, the large intestines began to drop on top of your pancreas. The more pounds you put in your colon, the more you began to crash the pancreas, slowing down the flow of insulin. So now your doctor is telling you to watch how much sugar you eat. The pancreas is what produces the insulin in your body. Let me give an example of what I'm saying, it's like me sitting on your pancreas for thirty years and every day I add 4 pounds. I will have crushed your pancreas to where it can't produce insulin any more, so now they're telling you that you're a diabetic and you cant have any more sugar. But you do have people that are borderline diabetics. That means there is not that much pressure on your pancreas, slowing down the insulin flow. Pressure from the larger colon and pressure from the large intestines will relieve some of the pressure off of your pancreas, making the insulin flow better. There is one thing you have to remember diabetes does not run in your family, it's just you all eat the same food causing the same problem. If it really ran in your family, why have you just been told that you have diabetes in your adult years? Think about it. If it ran in your family you would have had diabetes when you were born, it should be in your parents' blood.

Most people I talk to Say to me, why can't the doctor tell you what's really making your body go through so many new changes? Well, I am not a doctor but to me they are in the business for the money, not to help a person. That's why they never fix the problem. They sometimes just make it worse and cause more problems. But here are things you can do that will help you. Don't let the new pounds take over your body, making it hard for you to get around cause you're too heavy. Do not let it take over your mind where you think it's ok to be a little overweight or a lot overweight. Or you can become a guinea pig for your doctor to try new drugs on. You think this can help your weight problem, I don't think so, instead you just become bigger as the days go on.

Let me ask you a question. Since you have put on these new pounds, has it been hard for you to get around without breathing extra hard like you're about to pass out? How did it make you feel? I will let you think about it. How does it feel to know that you have to start living with this new weight? You're probably having a problem figuring out how you even got so big.

If out of nowhere you just started to gain weight did you ever stop to think that the dead animals you're eating carry pounds that will make you feel heavy? Well society nowadays thinks for the mass of people, and people just believe whatever they say. That's why few people know the truth about what's supposed to go in your body or that it is how much you put in your body that destroys the insides. People who have been heavy or overweight growing up are now used to having such breathing problems.

Many people carry around one of those inhalers, puffing every 5 minutes wishing they could get off the inhaler. The doctors have people thinking that they have asthma cause they do not know what to call it themselves. There are small-framed people who are using an inhaler because they have problems with their breathing too. However, there is more than one reason why your body needs extra oxygen. Asthma is a word the doctors made up, like many other words they have made up because they do not know what is really going on. When you have too much fat clogging up your organs that plays a big role in stopping your breathing. When one of your heart valves is not receiving all the oxygen it should get, this causes breathing problems.

The human body contains 70% percent water, which makes the blood run and keeps up the fluid level in the body. We have to put the other 30% of water into the body to keep your body going so you don't get dehydrated and pass out. When the doctor wants to give you information on oxygen, like telling you how to do CPR, CPR is good for every one to know because you never know when a person is going to need some oxygen to help them breathe. By breathing oxygen into a person, you give them some air to breathe into their lungs, which keeps them alive.

HEALTHY COLON

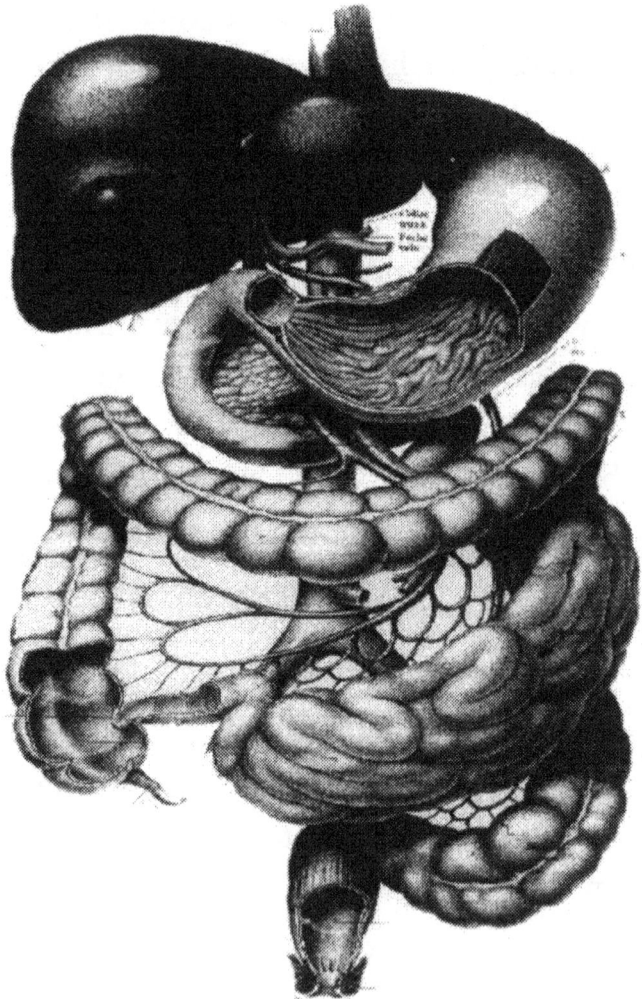

Fig. 1

Art from Anatomical Chart Company

24

UNHEALTHY COLON

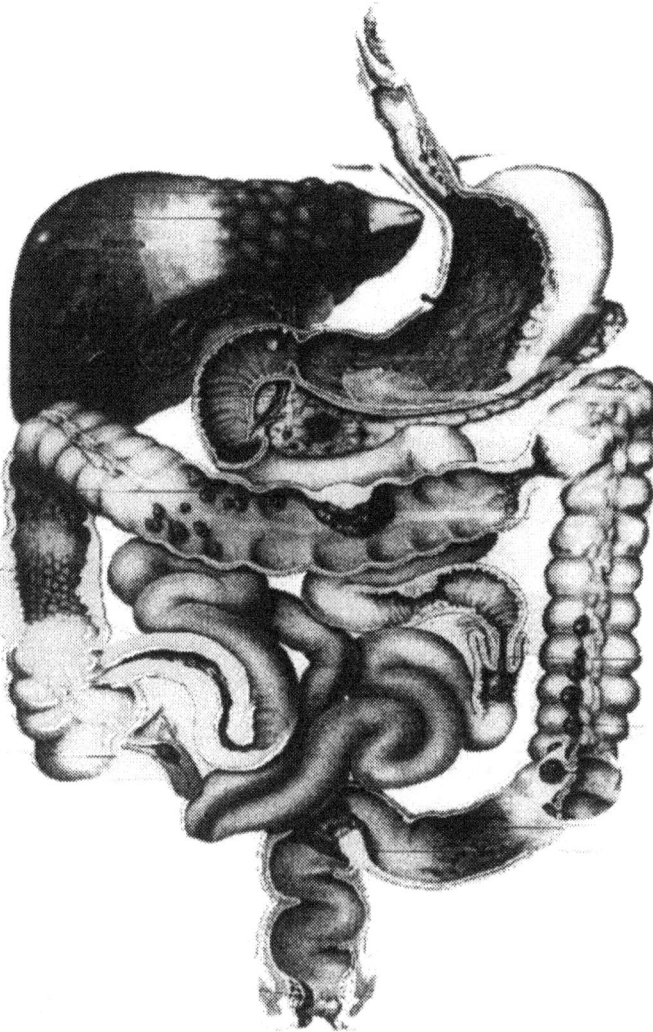

Fig. 2

Art from Anatomical Chart Company

Chapter 2

Where Is All This Fat Coming From?

Most people don't know that their body parts are made up of muscle tissue, not fatty tissue that covers your veins and other organs in the body. The fat on your body is like padding for your bones so they do not break as quickly when you injure yourself. Without fat the bone would break and fall off. The muscle is the padding for the fat; that is why the muscle tissue turns into fat once you stop using your muscles. So you have to maintain the growth of the muscle or it will turn into fatty tissue.

As soon as you start working out, the fat will turn back into muscle tissue. It's something like a tennis game, back and forth, back and forth. Some people only work out at the beginning of the year. Some just work out when they feel like working out so that is where the problem comes in. Do not forget that the muscle is not made of fat but it can turn into excess fatty tissue.

The human body works just like the car you are driving. Your car is made of a shell that we call a body, just like the human body. The main part that makes a car move is the battery; without the battery the car is dead. The main organs that make the body keep breathing are the lungs; without lungs the body is dead. You have to ask yourself why is the weight I have put on making my body break down faster by the day?

Well most people I talk to do not understand why GOD made your body to suffer; your body is really saying to them "please stop eating all that food, I can't take it any more." However, do you listen to your body and mind or to people that think their opinion is right? The person that's telling you that your weight looks good on you—is she or he just as big as you or the same as you? If they are, why are they trying to get smaller?

Most of the people that are overweight make themselves feel good about their weight problem, and it's easy to make someone feel good about their new size cause they're having problems losing it too. However, somewhere down the line you are thinking it is cool to weigh over a 100 pounds more than what your body can handle. Whatever is making you think that it's ok not to want to lose some of those new pounds that are wearing you down, I cannot understand?

Many people talk about how sluggish they feel after eating a meal or even after just eating a hamburger. When you eat meat, did you forget? Do you know just how many pounds of meat you can put in your body a day or even a week? Some people need to learn how to eat a small portion of food a day—a 5-ounce serving plus some vegetables is enough for most adults. One day you need to add up every pound of meat you eat, plus the muscle weight, and you will see just how big you will get. I know you may be saying to yourself there are people that eat meat and are not big-framed people. To tell you the truth, there is no one who was born to be an overweight person. The reason why you became overweight is because you just took in more food than a slim-framed person could take in.

Well, the meat you eat contains fat. Fat helps keep the body warm, but the extra fat you eat stores itself in the tissue. Body fat also works as food when your body is not getting enough food. If some one told you that you could only get protein by eating animal meat, they are dead wrong. You can get vegetable sources of protein from soybean and other products.

As I said earlier in the book, some people were fed too much food as babies and some just like to eat. What I am telling you is that your metabolism is what helps break down the food in your body. Now some people's metabolism is faster than other people's for example, a person who weighs 150 pounds, their body can normally only hold up to 5 or 10 pounds more than. Ok, their weight can fluctuate, but they will tend to weigh 150 pounds because of their metabolism helping to break down the food faster. Therefore, in this case the food does not clog up the rectum before it is ready to come out.

Now we have the people in the middle-weight category that weigh 210 pounds. They are usually solidly built (firm bodies). These type of bodies will never get too big or too small because they develop a solid frame with no cut or definition. Whatever weight they put on their bodies will keep them at the same weight, but they can add pounds to their colon to give them that big guy or big girl look.

Chapter 3

What Makes Your Colon So Big?

Well, earlier, I talked a little about the colon, how long it grows, and how many pounds you can put in the colon—up to 300 pounds without it ever coming out of the body. Once you start putting all that meat in your body, it makes it harder for the digestive system to work on getting it out of your body because the rectum is only so big and only so much can come out at a time.

Have you ever had a drainage problem with your sink? If you have, you can better understand what I'm talking about. If you put too much food in your sink, you can stop the sink up where only so much is coming out at a time. What do you do about it? Do you call a plumber or do you buy some liquid Drano to pour down your sink?

How would you unclog your sink or your colon? It will start to smell very badly in the area after a while and only so much can drain out at a time. The more you put in, the harder it makes it to go down. After a while, your sink will start to rot away. You will begin to have flies flying all around the sink because of the toxins that have built up in the area. This same thing happens to your colon; putting too much dead meat into your body will cause a toxin problem.

If the food you eat is not coming out the rectum correctly, it begins to rot inside of the body. Then in the end it begins to effect your liver and kidneys because those two organs are the filters of the body to get the toxins out of the body.

Then you start to worry about the new bad breath you have and the new body odor. Well, you're like a walking trash can. It doesn't matter how many times you clean the trashcan, it's still going to smell. You can brush your teeth three times a day and whenever you talk your breath is going to still stink.

The world we live in keeps people in a state of mind where they simply just don't pay attention to these types of things. The person next to you may smell the same way because they are eating the same thing you are eating. So people really do not think about it cause you are told that dead meat has protein so you may not think or believe it is the meat that causes it. Well, eat fruits and vegetables for a week or two and you will notice that you will not feel as sluggish after you have eaten a meal. Notice your breath will smell a lot different, your skin will start looking a lot healthier, and you will be full of energy. You can try it out for yourself and, believe me, you will love your new look and how you feel and your energy level.

My point is that you really can put on a different look. Have you ever seen a female who turned her colon into a pouch?

Wait, I may have gone over your head with that one about the colon and the pouch. Well, let me tell you a little about the colon and the pouch or the beer belly. Most people have not been told the truth about where the colon is, where the stomach is located, and what it has to do with the pouch. The mass of people I know have been told that their colon is their stomach. The stomach sits on the left side of the body. The stomach is right above the colon area, but they tell you it is in the middle of the body where some have a pouch or beer belly.

When you ask the average person where their stomach is, they will tell you under my rib cage and they will be pointing to their colon area. Yes, you are right, it is under your rib cage but to the left and on top of your colon, so how can it be in the front in what you call the pouch area? The stomach was not designed to store food; it's designed to break down the food with the help of your teeth, saliva and enzymes.

Why do the doctors have you thinking your colon area is the stomach area when it is not? By telling you that your colon is your stomach, they keep you in the dark. Is it so that you will never know the truth on how the colon will destroy your body organs? See, we all know that in order for the human body to survive we need food for energy. Somehow they'll have you think if your colon is filled up with too much food it will help you survive longer, but that's not your stomach, so what are you doing to yourself? I will give you a diagram of the location of the colon and the stomach. (See Fig. 3 on the following page you will find a diagram of the location of the colon and the stomach.)

Your stomach cannot hold that much food in it, in the first place, without bursting through your rib cage. That is why you have the liver and kidneys. Those two organs filter out the toxins in the colon. The stomach keeps the good stuff and sends the rest to the liver and kidney.

STOMACH and COLON

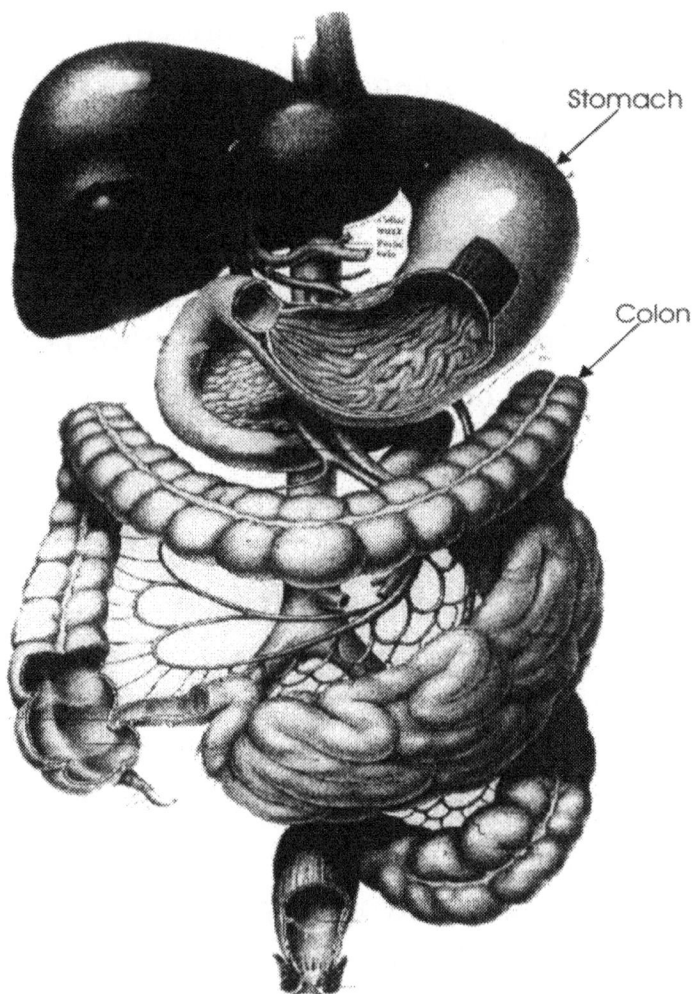

Fig. 3

Art from Anatomical Chart Company

The liver and kidney send the food to the colon where the colon stores the food while it goes through. It's a 24-hour breakdown system. Yes, it takes up to 24 hours to break down what you eat for the day from the morning to the evening. You want to be able to flush out the food by the next morning. This is just how your body works. This is something the doctor does not tell you.

If you have a slow metabolism it will make it harder for you to eliminate the food on the body's time cycle. What would happen is you would begin to take in more and more food. In addition, before you know it, you won't be able to look straight down at your feet cause the food will have started to clog up the rectum where it gets stuck and is now hard to come out.

As the days go by, if you are still eating big meals, you are compacting the colon, day in and day out, to make a pouch or beer belly. The more you compact your colon with all that food, the more pounds you are adding to your body.

Now remember I told you, your colon is like rubber, it just stretches and does not break. You can put up to 300 pounds in your colon and still live for a while, but your body will be like a truck sitting in a junkyard with only parts to pick from.

Chapter 4

What Happened To The Frame I Had?

By carrying those pounds around you are putting pressure on your organs, because they are not used to all that new pressure pushing up against them. If you look at a slim solid frame female or male you will notice that you can see their abdomen area (what you call the six pack). The abdomen muscle sits in front of your colon and protects your colon from physical harm. If someone stabbed a knife in your abdomen area, the knife wound have to be about 2 inches long depending on your size and how thick your muscle tissues are. The average person walking around today has forgotten that they even have abdominal muscles and how good they really look. What you have read today will help you learn about where your colon is, where the pounds go, and what is weight.

A lot of people talk about having problems with their abdomen area, giving them little sharp pains here and there, and not knowing where they're coming from. By filling your colon up with all that food, the 29-foot colon begins stretching and pushing right against your abdominal muscles, causing the pain. The colon is just a very strong organ and, when compacted, it becomes solid as a rock—it gets harder and harder. The only way to break up the solids you have made in your colon is to take a colon-cleansing product. When you start taking the colon cleanser, you will get relief from the pain.

You are emptying the weight and waste from those pounds you are holding. Some people think because they are getting bigger in the colon area that it is making them stronger, but it is really making them weaker. Their own weight and size fool some people. Then other people make them feel like they are stronger, just because of their size, by asking them to move things they know they can't move themselves. They can fool a lot of people this way but in the end there will always be the one who's really feeling left out cause they know they're weak, so they run when it comes to doing manual work. People cannot understand why the smaller framed person with the muscles can lift more weight than the bigger person.

The smaller person has not filled his colon with all those pounds. The slim framed person is straight up and down lean muscle, no extra fat or extra pounds in their colon weighing them down, taking away their physical strength. A middle framed or a large framed person, who is carrying over 50 to 100 pounds extra weight, is like walking around with a 40-pound weight around your neck, and Wondering why you are feeling so sluggish. The only way to drop some of the pounds and get your strength back is by flushing the pounds out of your colon.

When you start to take a colon cleanser, you do not have to worry about depending on the product your entire life. The colon product is not a drug; it's made from herbs so there are no side effects. Prescription drugs are the only things you can take to heal your body that make your body depend on them. Doctors want you to take prescription drugs. They do not know if the drugs are really going to work; that's why when one doesn't work they give you another one to try or they add more milligrams.

Now you're complaining to your doctor about how the drug is not working for your body. They tell you that you must not be taking the drugs cause they work for everybody, but you're not everybody. Why don't they just tell you that they want you to try this drug to see if it works for you?

Now you may hear a lot about herbs; people may give you testimonies on how well herbs are working for them. However, you still cannot believe that herbs really work because

50

your doctor is telling you they do not know much about herbs so just keep taking the drugs. However, the drugs they are making and giving you are made with chemicals so you do not really know what you are getting; that is why you are having side effects.

Herbs come from a natural source—from plants. They are meant to heal the body from toxins and poisons that enter the body. Most people from the south had grandparents that made them drink castor oil after every meal. Why? Because they knew after killing an animal the dead animal becomes poison, so you have to clean it quick, then cook it, and then get the poison out of your body. As soon as you eat the animal you want to flush it out.

When you are cooking the meat in grease, the poison is now flowing in your pan. Then you save the grease and cook with it again, how nasty! If you have never steamed or gril-led your food, try it and notice how much extra grease and fat will run out. I know you are looking for good Physical health but you have to listen to your own mind and try what works for you and what can help your body, and not what you have heard others say.

After a while, the colon starts to effect many of your organs because of the many pounds you put in your colon without flushing out the waste.

One of the first questions I ask a person is, how many times a day do they have a bowel elimination. Most people say they have elimination once or twice a day and some only go three-four times a week, which is not good at all. The average person should have a bowel elimination after every meal. However, most people eat, all through the day, junk food and fast foods.

Chapter 5

How The Food Is Digested Through The Body

Human bodies only need to take in three nice-sized meals a day. You should balance your meals with proteins, vegetables, fruits, breads and dairy. Remember to drink eight 8 oz. glass of water per day. Drink your liquids 30 minutes before or 30 minutes after your meal.

The esophagus takes 10 second to mix food with saliva before passing it through the esophagus into the stomach.

The liver produces a green liquid called bile to help break down fats in the food. Then the kidneys filter water and urea from the blood and expel the mixture as urine.

The urine travels from the kidney along the urethra into the bladder. The bladder stores the urine and when the bladder is full it contracts to push the urine out of the body.

The pancreas makes juices, which convert carbohydrates, protein and fats into chemical mixtures used by the body. (The small intestine's digestive juices that's produced in the liver, pancreas and small intestine break down the food). (Takes up to 4-5 hours to pass through)

Water and undigested food pass into the large intestine. (Takes up to 7-16 hours to pass the food through)

The solid waste from the large intestines is stored in the rectum. The anus muscle is what pushes the solid waste out of the anus as feces. This is how the food breaks down in the body. This may help you understand how your bodies work. It is possible for you to create a new body for yourself, start today.

BOOK AVAILABLE THROUGH

Milligan Books, Inc.

An Imprint of Professional Business Consulting Service

**ARE WEIGHT AND POUNDS
THE SAME THING? $12.00**

Order Form

Milligan Books, Inc.

1425 W. Manchester Ave., Suite C, Los Angeles, CA 90047

(323) 750-3592

Name_____ Date _____

Address

City_____ State____ Zip Code _____

Day Telephone _____

Evening Telephone_____

Book Title_____

Number of books ordered___ Total.........$ _____

Sales Taxes (CA Add 8.25%) ....$ _____

Shipping & Handling $3.90 for one book..$ _____

Add $1.00 for each additional book..........$ _____

Total Amount Due...............................$ _____

☐ Check   ☐ Money Order ☐ Other Cards _____

☐ Visa   ☐ MasterCard Expiration Date _____

Credit Card No. _____

Driver License No. _____

Make check payable to Milligan Books, Inc.

_____   _____

Signature   Date